Long COVID Treatments

To Do At Home

Right Now

by Charles Kilmer

ISBN 9798390533215

Design by *Veronika Grebennikova*

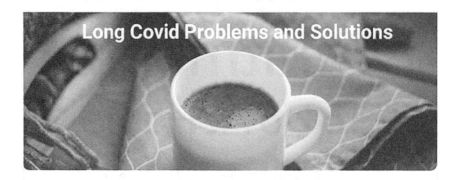

Long Covid Problems and Solutions

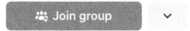

Join the evolving conversation about your symptoms at **Long COVID Problems and Solutions** https://www.facebook.com/groups/longcovidproblemsandsolutions/.

Table of Contents

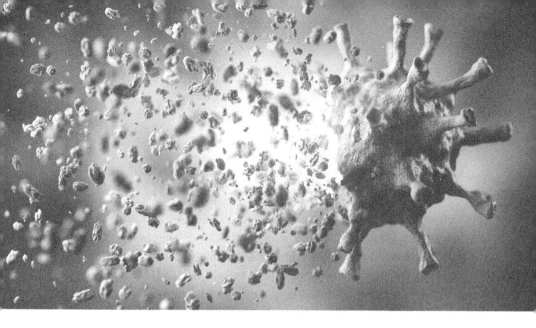

Introduction

The outbreak of COVID-19 pandemic changed the world. COVID-19 created unprecedented challenges for everyone. One of the long-lasting impacts of the pandemic is Long COVID.

Over 600 million people have contracted COVID-19. Over 6 million people have died.[1] Some people have lingering effects of the disease. These lingering effects of COVID are called Long COVID.

Most long COVID patients have preexisting conditions. These pre-conditions include autoimmune[2] and chronic diseases. Pre-existing conditions also include allergies—even virus's patients once had. Mold and mildew can provoke long COVID. There are other risk factors for Long COVID. These risk factors include poverty, smoking, obesity, and type 2 diabetes. Dark skin in northern latitudes poses a risk. Because dark skin does not absorb sunlight very well. (More on that later.)

These preconditions make the body vulnerable to long COVID.

No one treatment will solve the problem. Instead, this book offers layer upon layer of treatments. These treatments, taken together, offer the best chance for success.

Are you one of those suffering from the effects of your bout with COVID? Are you looking for answers?

We offer a practical guide to good health and a return to a normal life.

The Lingering Effects of COVID-19: Understanding the Prevalence and Impact of Long COVID

Long COVID is also known as chronic COVID and long-haul COVID. Some other names are post-acute COVID-19 or long-term COVID. The current official name for long COVID is post-acute sequelae SARS-CoV-2 infection (PASC).[3]

The Center for Disease Control (CDC) says Long COVID is not one singular health issue. Rather, long COVID is a group of health problems. These problems occur after recovering from COVID-19. They can last weeks, months, or even years.[4]

As of July 2021, the US government escalated the status of Long COVID. It is now a disability under the Americans with Disabilities Act (ADA).[5] England offers employment compensation by way of the Personal Independence Payment.

On the bright side, for many, Long COVID symptoms can improve over time. But for some, Long COVID can last for months and escalate into a chronic health condition. For these folk, the Americans with Disabilities Act will be very helpful.

The Varied and Evolving Symptoms of Long COVID

When the CDC first reported Long COVID, there were around 8 symptoms. Now there are over 200.[6] Each person has different symptoms. That makes treatment difficult.

We highlight and group below some of the primary symptoms of Long COVID.

A Closer Look at the Most Common Symptoms of Long COVID

- Fever

- Symptoms get worse after physical or mental effort. This is "post-exertional malaise, or PEM")
- Fatigue or tiredness that affects daily life

Respiratory and Heart Symptoms
- Heart Palpitations
- Chest pain
- Cough
- Difficulty breathing or shortness of breath

Neurological Symptoms
- Difficulty concentrating or thinking (brain fog)
- Headache
- Change in taste or smell
- Dizziness when you stand up (lightheadedness)
- Pins-and-needles feelings
- Depression or anxiety
- Sleep problems

Digestive Symptoms
- Stomach pain
- Diarrhea

Other Symptoms
- Changes in menstrual cycles
- Joint or muscle pain
- Rash

The Science behind Long COVID: What We Know and What We're Still Learning

Fifty percent of the people who go to the hospital with COVID-19 end up with Long COVID.[7] Many people catch COVID-19 but don't go to the hospital. Of these people roughly 20% have some kind of illness that lasts for months—or longer.[8] Sometimes the problems are small—like the loss of smell. Other times, people may suffer from a lack of willpower to do anything. Some people have become paralyzed. They are unable to get out of bed because they have no energy. They can't handle any amount of physical or mental stress.

The symptoms may go away. Patients may feel good for a while. They may think they're moving forward. But then the old symptoms return. They feel even worse. Failure to improve creates a sense of despair and a lack of hope.

For many people, just making ends meet becomes a problem because they can no longer work. The stress of being unable to work triggers their symptoms.

The old are most vulnerable to COVID-19. Yet, Long COVID does not affect the old so much. On average, it affects people who are 43 and in their prime. Both men and women get COVID-19, but the demographics of Long COVID skew toward women.[9]

What causes long COVID? There is good evidence that COVID-19 debris or the COVID-19 virus itself causes long COVID.

There is currently a worldwide community of Long COVID sufferers. This book draws from the wisdom of this community. You can join the evolving conversation about your symptoms at Long COVID Problems and Solutions.

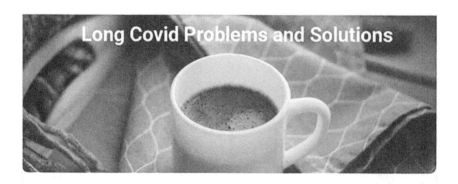

Long Covid Problems and Solutions

This book will bring you the information you need — to know how to feel better and get better at home.

Fighting Long COVID: Our Solutions

We will give you many actionable solutions. Take the steps provided in the order that we provide them. Each step leads to another step which leads to better health.

We will talk about in order

1. Test and treat for histamine intolerance.[10]
2. Then we will talk about the body and its' innate immune system. Many of us have frail immunity. COVID-19 preyed on those frailties and settled in to take over.[11] The goal will be to try different treatments to restore the strength of your innate immune system. Our innate immune system becomes stronger when given layer upon layer of treatments
3. For much of Chapter 1 and succeeding chapters we will talk about lowering stress. Stress is what most often sets off the worst symptoms of long COVID.[12]

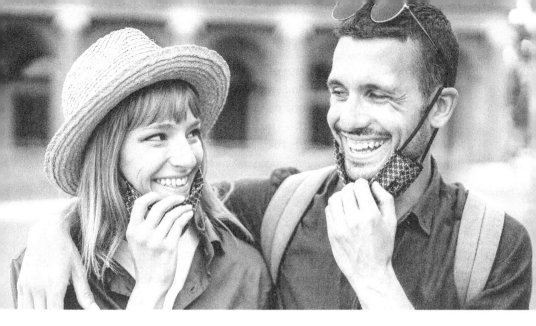

Chapter 1:
Four Things to do Right Now

This chapter focuses on the steps you can take **right now** to combat Long COVID. These steps include:

- Buy an antihistamine[13]
- Learn how to do a low antihistamine diet for a couple of weeks.[14]
- Learn the importance of Nicotinamide Adenine Dinucleotide (NAD$^+$)[15] and Glutathione.[16] These molecules strengthen your body's ability to heal and defend itself. Glutathione is the cornerstone of your body's immune system. NAD$^+$ increase your body's production of energy. This energy enables glutathione to do its work.
- There will be recommendations for lowering stress.

Start a Low Histamine Diet

It is important that we discuss mast cells before we get into the benefits of a low histamine diet. Mast cells are a type of white blood cell that causes many of the symptoms of Long COVID.[17] Allergens or toxins cause allergic and inflammatory responses in these cells. Allergens or toxins live in our tissues and organs. Mast Cell Activation Syndrome (MCAS) is a health problem. MCAS affects people with auto-immune diseases.

Scientists think that COVID-19 may also cause MCAS.[18] When a person has MCAS, the mast cells overreact. They create too much histamine. This histamine triggers severe allergy reactions in various body organs. These body organs include the heart and the respiratory system. MCAS can also take place in the gastrointestinal tract and the skin.[19]

What is Histamine?

The mast cells in our body make histamine,[20] but histamines are also found in foods.[21] They activate the immune system to fight off bacteria and viruses.[22]

Most of us tolerate histamine in foods. But some people don't have diamine oxidase, an enzyme that breaks down histamine in foods.[23] This can lead to a person having too much histamine, leading to histamine intolerance.

According to WebMD, "approximately 1% of the population has a histamine intolerance.[24] For these people, histamine builds up in the body and is not broken down. This can trigger an immune system response…."

Histamine intolerance can cause diarrhea, heart palpitations, and asthma. Histamine intolerance can cause low blood pressure, runny nose, headaches and nasal congestion. For some people, these symptoms can last for a few hours up to a few days when they take a meal high in histamine.[25]

Some long COVID symptoms and histamine intolerance symptoms are very similar. Some doctors think that there may be a link.[26]

Histamine Intolerance Diagnosis

There are many auto immune diseases. These include multiple sclerosis (MS), rheumatoid arthritis (RA), and bullous pemphigoid. But there are many more. People with any auto-immune diseases may suffer from long COVID histamine intolerance.[27]

Do you have an auto immune disease?

The problem with diagnosing histamine intolerance is that there are no simple tests for it.[28] Food allergy tests do not work because histamine intolerance is not a food allergy. As a result, the first recommendation is to rule out histamine intolerance. This happens by avoiding foods high in histamine.[29]

The best way to start the low histamine diet is the elimination diet.[30] Elimination diet is a meal plan where you cut foods causing health issues. In this case, we're talking about foods high in histamines.

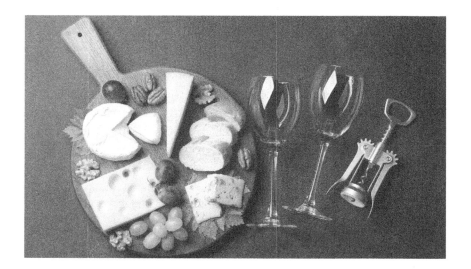

Foods High in Histamine[31]

Here are basic foods that have high levels of histamine you should avoid:
- Nuts:
- Peanuts
- Tree nuts
- Beer and wine
- Vegetables: tomatoes spinach,
- Fruits: bananas oranges
- Processed meats
- Cured meats
- Fermented dairy such as aged cheese
- Pickled, fermented, or tinned fish

Fresh fruits and vegetables have less histamine. Canned food, fermented food, or food stored for long periods have more. The longer food sits out, gets stored, or aged, the more histamine it contains.

Let's break down the high histamine foods into groups and take a closer look.

Fermented Foods

Sauerkraut is usually a healthy fermented food. It is high in vitamin C but has very high histamine concentrations compared to other foods.

Alcohol

Alcohol increases histamine levels. The reaction to histamines in alcohol can cause migraines.

Packaged Meat

Packaged, preserved, or smoked meats contain high levels of histamine. According to WebMD, histamine levels differ between meats depending on the cooking process. Grilling meat increases histamine level, and boiling reduces it.

Aged Cheese

Cheese needs a cool stable temperature for long-term preservation. Unstable temperature affects histamine levels in cheese.

Legumes

Legumes, like peanuts or chickpeas, can cause major allergic reactions in asthma patients.

Citrus Fruit

Citrus fruit itself doesn't contain much histamine. But they can trigger the release of histamine in the body. For a test—try taking citrus fruit out of your diet for a brief period of time.

Low Histamine Foods[32]

The following six foods have low histamine levels.
- Whole grain products, including bread and pasta
- Herbal tea but not green or black tea
- Fresh vegetables leafy greens, parsley, onions, cabbage, arugula, broccoli and many more.
- Fresh fruit: plantains, kiwi, blackberries
- Fresh meat
- Coconut milk and rice

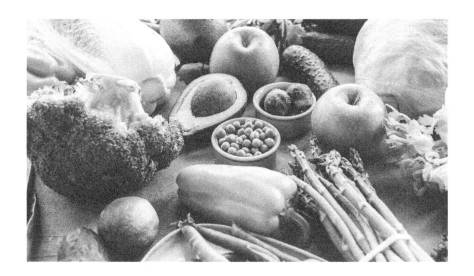

Low Histamine Diet Challenges[33]

Lack of willpower

Staying on a low histamine diet is especially challenging for Long COVID patients. Often Long COVID sufferers lack the willpower to stay on a restrictive diet.

Finding a dietician

Consider a visit to a registered dietician. Ask the dietician or doctor if lowering your histamine levels is a good choice. A dietician can help during the restrictive phase of the diet. At the right time, they can help re-introduce histamine foods into the diet.

You may need to choose a doctor or dietician. Choose wisely. Ask them about Mast Cell Activation Syndrome or histamine intolerance. They should be aware of this condition. If not, go elsewhere.

The Timing of Your Diet: How Long Should You Stick to It?

The other thing to note is that this diet should be short-term in most cases.

Try the low histamine diet for two to four weeks. If there is no change, your problem is not high histamine levels. If you are not better after two to four weeks, re-introduce high histamine foods into your diet.

Medicines and Histamine Intolerance

Ask your doctor or healthcare professional about your medicines. Check the brands you take for their histamine tolerances.

Buying Antihistamines Over the Counter[34]

As you start the low histamine diet, go to your local drug store and buy antihistamines. (If you have a history of problems with antihistamines—don't take them.)

Generations of antihistamines

The first generation:

The oldest group of over-the-counter (OTC) antihistamines is the first generation. These original antihistamines make you drowsy. They also don't last long in your system. First-generation brands include Chlor-Trimeton and Benadryl.

The second and third generation:

These generations of antihistamines won't make you drowsy. They work longer. So, you don't have to take many doses. Examples of these brands are Allegra, Claritin, and Zyrtec.

Take the second and third-generation non-drowsy antihistamines in the morning. Take the first-generation antihistamines in the evening. The first-generation antihistamines tend to cause drowsiness.

Natural Histamine Blocker

You may not be able to go to the pharmacy and buy an antihistamine. Do you have a histamine intolerance? There are natural supplement that you can take which degrade histamines.[35] These include:

- Stinging Nettle
- Vitamin C
- Quercetin
- Butterbur
- Bromelain
- Probiotics
- Diamine Oxidase[36]

Low Dose Naltrexone

Do you have both long COVID and autoimmune disease? There is an inexpensive drug called Naltrexone. It can help with brain fog, shortness of breath, heart arrhythmia and hypertension. Take low doses of this drug.[37]

Ivermectin

Ivermectin is another low cost solution for some of the symptoms of long COVID. These symptoms include muscle pain, fatigue, sleep, memory and mood issues.

Recent Ivermectin tests showed a 72% reduction in laboratory-confirmed infections. The drug also showed no severe side effects.

Not all can take ivermectin. Some may be allergic and it may cause side effects such as nausea, dizziness, and chest discomfort. It's important to consult a healthcare provider before taking Ivermectin.

Both Ivermectin and low dose naltrexone show promise. They can resolve some of the symptoms of long COVID. Try both. If one doesn't work. Try the other.[38]

What they don't do is strengthen the body's underlying innate immune system. That only happens by increasing your body to youthful levels of glutathione and NAD$^+$.

We will discuss glutathione and NAD$^+$ in the next section.

The Adaptive vs. Innate Immune System

COVID vaccinations focus on the adaptive immune system.[39] The adaptive immune system is the part of our body that fights foreign proteins. These include colds, flu, and COVID-19. The adaptive immune system develops B cells and T cells. These cells fight against foreign proteins.[40]

But the adaptive immune system is the second line of defense. The first line of defense for your body is the innate or nonspecific immune system.[41] You are born with the innate immune system. Children have strong innate immune systems. Their innate immune system protects them against viruses.[42] Innate immunity presents barriers that keep harmful viruses -from disrupting your body. These harmful viruses include colds, flus and COVID. We will next be focusing on this first line of defense.

Why?

Auto immune and chronic diseases weaken or misguide the innate immune system. Even mold and mildew will weaken your innate immune system. Age itself weakens your innate immune system. Weakened innate immune systems make you more vulnerable to COVID and long COVID.

But people with a strong innate immune system are less susceptible to either COVID or long COVID.[43] This is the reason that children are relatively immune from COVID. Children have strongest innate immune systems.[44]

So, one goal of this book is to show you the treatments that strengthen your innate immune system.

A strong innate immune system is the body's ultimate armor against disease. This part of the immune system doesn't care what the COVID variant is. The innate immune system fights the virus without targeting a specific spike protein.[45]

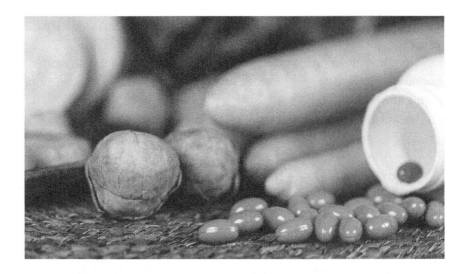

Long COVID supplements

NAD+

Many Long COVID patients often complain of low energy levels. This is likely because of low Nicotinamide Adenine Dinucleotide (NAD+) levels.[46] NAD+ is the molecule responsible for Adenosine Triphosphate (ATP) production. ATP is the fuel of mitochondria.

Mitochondria are the energy powerhouses of your body and its cells. ATP is what gives the mitochondria their power. ATP gives us the power to get out of bed in the morning and do all the things we do all day long.[47]

NAD+ is critical for maintaining healthy ATP levels.

Loss of NAD+ can cause age-related diseases.[48] These include loss of strength, frailty, metabolic disease, cancer, and cognitive decline.

NAD+ decreases naturally with age. The rate of decline of NAD+ can speed up. Type II diabetes, autoimmune diseases, and chronic illness can hasten the loss of NAD+.[49]

The above problems diminish NAD+ levels. Long COVID can further deplete your NAD+.[50] That's why you have no energy. So this next section is about how you can restore your NAD+ levels.

NMN

NMN is an NAD+ precursor. This also converts to NAD+. NMN is a variant of Vitamin B3. NMN enables your body to make energy for everything you do.

NMN is fat-soluble, not water-soluble, meaning if you take it by mouth, you must mix it with olive oil or yogurt. You can also take it under the tongue. Or 2 grams mixed with olive oil or yogurt. Store in the refrigerator.

Trimethylglycine TMG[51]

TMG restores methyls metabolized by NMN. Take 2 grams of TMG daily.

Leucine

Leucine improves the body's ability to absorb NMN. Take 4 grams daily.

Apigenin[52]

Apigenin prevents an enzyme called CD-38 from destroying NAD+ in the body. This is as important as taking NAD+ precursors to increase your NAD+. So, you should take an apigenin supplement with NAD+ boosters. Mix apigenin with either olive oil or yogurt. Store in the refrigerator.

Parsley, celery, and chamomile tea are foods high in apigenin.[53] Dried parsley is cheap. 500 mg of parsley in capsules is also cheap. The amount of chamomile tea you'd need to take is impractical. Instead, take 500 mg of parsley and 50 mg of apigenin supplement daily.

Increase Glutathione Levels

Long COVID patients tend to suffer from pre-existing health issues. These include various autoimmune or chronic diseases. These also include weight-related challenges, pre-diabetes, or Type II diabetes. These health challenges create a problem for Long COVID sufferers. These pre-existing conditions reduce Glutathione levels in the body.

Glutathione levels decline with age.[54] Autoimmune diseases and chronic diseases further reduce the body's store of glutathione.[55] Extra visceral fat around the tummy causes oxidative stress. That reduces the body's store of glutathione.[56] COVID and Long COVID can wipe out most of whatever remains of the body's glutathione.

With no glutathione, there is no resistance to infection. Simple health issues can escalate fast.[57]

The liver produces glutathione. Glutathione is a combination of the amino acids glycine, cysteine, and glutamic acid. Glutathione helps builds tissue and repairs them. Glutathione makes the chemicals and proteins needed for immune system function. Glutathione enables Vitamin D to do its job.[58]

Like NAD+, glutathione is part of the innate immune system. Glutathione is not bioavailable. You can't take glutathione alone because it doesn't absorb well through the stomach. You can increase glutathione levels with glycine and n-acetyl cysteine (NAC).[59] Its also helpful to add a small amount of l-serine.[60]

If you have an autoimmune, chronic disease—or you're +65—start with a very high dose of NAC and glycine.[61] This would be 4 grams each of glycine and N-Acetyl L-Cysteine or NAC. Do that twice daily. For best results, include a third precursor of l- serine[62] in smaller doses. Take 200–500 mg once daily.

Glycine and l serine have no side effects. For some people high dose NAC can cause stomach upset. So start off with one gram of NAC. Then build up from there.

Take NAC and Glycine at high levels for a month. After a month, scale that back to 3 grams each of glycine and NAC twice daily. If you have a chronic disease, auto immune disease or type 2 diabetes—maintain those levels. If you have none of those factors, drop your dosages to 2 grams each of glycine and NAC twice daily.

There is one caution. Long COVID can cause micro clots in the blood. Blood thinners will defend against micro clots. NAC in high doses is a mild blood thinner. NAC will give some defense against micro clots in the blood.

This is good for COVID sufferers. But, if you're already taking a blood thinner like coumadin—you should consult with your doctor. This is less of an issue if you're taking 81 mg baby aspirin. A baby aspirin is not a powerful blood thinner.

Vitamin D

Vitamin D is a fat-soluble vitamin. Vitamin D is not a vitamin. It's a hormone. Vitamin D helps the body absorb calcium and phosphorus. Both are critical for building bone. Vitamin D can reduce cancer cell growth, help control infections and reduce inflammation. Vitamin D is in every cell of the body. Vitamin D is involved with both the adaptive and innate immune system.[63] Vitamin D helps fight off COVID. People with autoimmune disease usually have low levels of vitamin D.

Its important to take glutathione to increase your body's ability to absorb Vitamin D. Its also important to take Vitamin D.

A daily dose of 30K International Units (IU) should be enough to start with. Long COVID patients with pre-existing conditions should consider higher doses. These pre-existing conditions include type II diabetes, autoimmune or chronic diseases. If you don't have the pre-existing conditions start with 10k iu.

Get a blood test after a month to check your Vitamin D level and adjust your dose. Aim for the optimal 60–80 ng ml Vitamin D level.[64]

We will talk more about Vitamin D later.

Lower Stress

The global reaction to COVID-19 created a high level of stress. At first, most governments demanded and enforced lockdowns. The COVID-19 lockdowns and social distancing disrupted social norms. They forced people to acclimate to a new normal. The isolation contributed to many sad outcomes. These included a high suicide rate.[65] People need human contact. Human contact is essential for maintaining mental health and well-being.

Science shows that when a person is under stress for long periods of time, their immune system weakens.[66]

The body when stressed, dumps the hormones adrenalin and cortisol into the bloodstream. Adrenaline increases heart rate, blood pressure, and energy supplies. Cortisol increases blood sugar levels and enhances brain glucose use and tissue repair.[67]

Cortisol and adrenaline are good for short periods of time. They help, especially in dangerous situations. This gives a person the boost of energy needed to address the danger. It's called the fight or flight response. [68]

Cortisol and adrenaline may be bad for you if you're stressed for too long. Staying in fight or flight mode for days, weeks, months, or even years wears out the body.[69]

Today, stress comes from many different parts of life. Stress can come from work, commutes, home, and school. Stress can come from anywhere and everywhere. Rather than burning off stress, most of us live with it. Stress is a constant reality of our active lives.[70]

Long COVID can cut the body's ability to deal with stress. Stress sets off the symptoms of Long COVID. Long COVID can make a person feel too weak or absorbed with Long COVID issues to do their normal chores. The inability to do normal chores further stresses people out. It can be a vicious cycle.[71]

Listed below are the proven ways to lower your stress level.

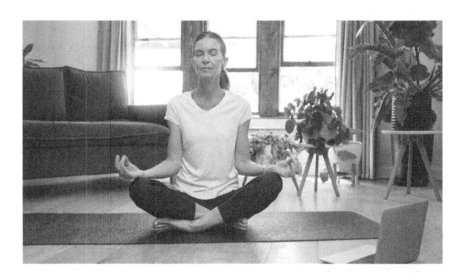

Meditation

Meditation is a proven way to reduce stress.[72] Meditation also helps with concentration and improves sleep. More sleep provides real results on both the physical and psychological levels.

Meditation also helps us to be more productive during the day.[73] Meditation teaches us how to be more present in the moment.[74]

You may think meditation is an odd practice. You may think meditation involves people doing strange things. That would be wrong.

What is Meditation?

Meditation is the process of quieting the mind. The average human being has around 6,000 thoughts per day.[75] Too many thoughts are of worry, fear or negative self-talk.

Meditation helps to stop the barrage of negative thoughts. Meditation causes the body and mind to be in sync. This sync stops the negative thoughts and fears. When the human heart and brain are in harmony, the body becomes calmer, more peaceful, and more mindful.[76] Meditation lowers stress.

How to Meditate

Start by finding a place where you can be alone for 15 to 20 minutes. Make sure you have taken care of any personal needs beforehand. Find a way to be comfortable during the session.

Get a timer or use one from your phone and set it for 15 minutes.
- Find a comfortable chair and sit upright in it. You can lie down on the floor or a bed. But you risk falling asleep if you choose to lay on your back or stomach.
- Close your eyes. If you cannot keep your eyes closed, get an eye mask and place it over your eyes.

In your room, listen for the sound of a fan, a washing machine, the air conditioner or any mundane sound. The goal is to find a quiet sound that may help you to focus on something other than your thoughts.

Next, focus on that sound and give your mind a break. Try not to think of anything. One of the first roadblocks is that thoughts will start coming into your mind. It's not a matter of if they will come. It's a matter of when.

Allow those thoughts in your mind to float by or think of them as floats going by in a parade. Even for experienced meditators, thoughts come up, so allow them to come and go. Part of the experience may include the feeling of numbness in your arms and legs.

So, when you do have this feeling, do not worry. That is normal. It means that your mind has transitioned into a deep state of consciousness. This is a good thing because it is where the psychological and physical benefits are.

When the timer goes off your session has ended. Open your eyes and turn off the alarm. Bask in the feeling of tranquility and peace. If you find it difficult to meditate for 15 minutes, start with five and work your way up. If you cannot meditate every day, start by meditating twice a week. Worrying about anything while meditating is counterproductive. Do not worry about doing it the right way.[77]

There are excellent guided meditation videos on YouTube. You can make use of the meditation apps available for download. Guided meditation has the benefit of keeping your mind occupied. You will focus on what the narrator says. You'll spend less time adrift.

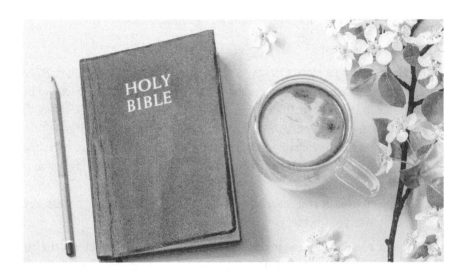

Prayer

For those who believe in God, prayer also lowers stress, improves sleep, and helps you feel better.

Photosonix

There are tools available which will train your mind to the state you desire. You may want to meditate, or concentrate, or sleep, or visualize the future, or relax. The machine will use headphones and glasses to deliver sight and sound to your mind. These sights and sounds together mimic the brainwaves that are characteristic of meditation, concentration or sleep. There are several companies that have this tool. One recommended here is by Photosonix. Be sure to read carefully the warnings that come with the product. [78]

Talk to a friend

Talking to a friend can help reduce stress because people are social creatures. We need one another to feel connected, loved, and appreciated.[79]

But, only positive friends can help you become better. Choose positive friends who lift you up, not drag you down.[80] That also means that you cannot drag your friends down either. Even though it is tempting, do not transfer negative energy to your friends. Do your best to stay positive. Long COVID symptoms might make you feel awful. But do your best to remain positive no matter how bad things are.[81]

Sending text messages is fine if you feel like you don't have the energy to manage phone calls. It may be challenging to maintain long-distance relationships. Online communities are also helpful.

You can join a facebook community for support and advice. Go to facebook groups and type in: "Long COVID Problems and Solutions" in the search bar. When the result pops up, join the group **Long COVID Problems and Solutions** at https://www.facebook.com/groups/longcovidproblemsandsolutions/.

As well, here is a list of Long COVID groups outside of Facebook.
- National Patient Advocate Foundation. COVID Care Resource Center[82]
- Body Politic COVID-19 Support Group[83]

Take walks outside

Get out and take a walk whenever you can. Walking can revitalize your spirit. Walks help you to de-stress.

Regular walks help your cardiovascular system.[84] Walking is healthy and great for your legs and calf muscles. Walking is one way to avoid varicose veins and swelling in the lower legs.[85] Walking can help you cut your Long COVID stress.[86]

If you live in a concrete jungle, walking is still an excellent choice to relieve stress. Walk in the park near trees, or find greenery that you can look at. Plants need sunlight for photosynthesis. The human body needs sunlight for optimal health.[87] A walk in the park for half an hour a day can do wonders to raise your spirits and lower stress.[88]

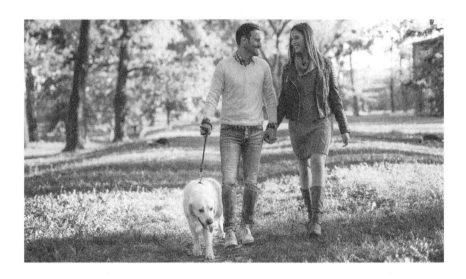

Walk Bare Feet or Buy a Grounding Mat

In 2010 a book was released called Earthing. The book showed the health benefits of walking barefoot. The book showed that living in contact with the Earth's natural surface charge—being grounded—naturally discharges and reduces chronic inflammation in the body. Chronic inflammation is one of the primary source of vulnerability to long COVID.

The US National Institute of Health confirmed the claims of the book.

Grounding appears to:

1. improve sleep.
2. normalize the day–night cortisol rhythm
3. reduce pain
4. reduce stress
5. shift the autonomic nervous system from sympathetic toward parasympathetic activation
6. increase heart rate variability
7. speed wound healing
8. reduce blood viscosity[89]

No need to go barefoot in the park. You can just buy a grounding mat on amazon. Then plug it in. That will replicate the effects of walking barefoot in the grass.

Get a pet

If you have ever wanted a pet, this is the perfect excuse to get one! Pets are great because they offer unconditional love and excellent companionship. A dog will get you up and out the door and help you move more often. Hospitals sometimes use pet therapy. Animals are good at making patients feel better. People who feel better heal faster. Pets lower stress.[90]

Cats are also good for healing and need less work than a dog.[91] This can be good, depending on your schedule and your current exercise regime. Get a cat if you're too busy for a dog, but don't relent on exercise. Many animal shelters have wonderful cats and dogs. They'd love for you to bring one home. Pets from an animal shelter can be well-behaved when they get adopted. Do your research before adopting any type of pet to be sure you are getting the pet most suitable for you.

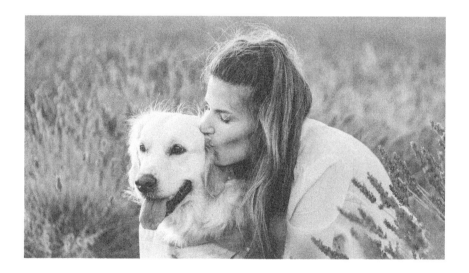

There are other pet choices. These include birds, hamsters, and rodents. For most people, these smaller pets will not provide much companionship. So they won't provide much relief from stress.[92]

Stop Watching The News[93]

Watching the news was once informative. News helped us learn about the world. But the world has changed. News has become secondary. The media now instill fear into people to increase their ratings. Fear is not healthy for anyone.[94] Living in fear wreaks havoc on the immune system.[95]

But fear sells.

For example, traffic slows down as it passes a car wreck on the side of the road. People are not being cautious because of the wreck. They are only rubbernecking to see what terrible thing happened. That's modern media— a constant wreck to keep you rubbernecking.

That's good for the news business but bad for your health.

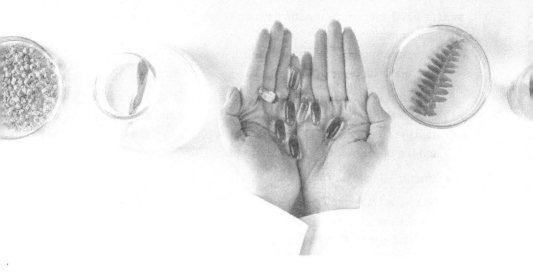

Chapter 2:

Change your body chemistry

C hanging your body chemistry can set you up for improved health. Yes, you can change your body chemistry. You can do that with vitamins, minerals, sunlight, oxygen therapy, and food. We will cover these options in this chapter.

Long COVID supplements

Many supplements can improve the health and well being of Long COVID sufferers. But, only in cases where you are severely lacking in a vitamin or mineral will these supplements have a noticeable effect on your symptoms. In most cases, these supplements will not alter your symptoms. Rather, they will strengthen your underlying innate immune system.

So why take them if they don't give an immediate benefit? Because COVID is like the flue. It changes. COVID evolves. So, there's no such thing as herd immunity. COVID wants to find a weak point in your innate immune system—and attack it. You want a strong innate immune system so to resist further reinfection.

Here is a Long COVID supplement list:

- **Selenium:** 100mcg / day[96]

  Selenium is an essential component of various enzymes and proteins, called selenoproteins, that help to make DNA and protect against cell damage and infections; these proteins are also involved in reproduction and the metabolism of thyroid hormones.

- **Zinc:** 15–30mg / day[97]

  Zinc is a trace mineral. That means that the body only needs small amounts of zinc. Yet zinc is necessary for almost 100 enzymes to carry out vital chemical reactions. It is a major player in the creation of DNA and the growth of cells. Zinc helps build proteins , heal damaged tissue, and supports a healthy immune system.

- **Quercetin:** 500mg 3x / day[98]

  Quercetin strengthens the innate immune system. It does this by increasing the production and activity of natural killer cells. Natural killer are a type of white blood cell. Natural killer cells help the body recognize and destroy virus-infected cells. Also, Quercetin has anti-inflammatory properties. Quercetin can help reduce the inflammation that can occur as a result of an infection or injury. Quercetin helps the body fight off pathogens and speeds up the healing process.

- **Vitamin C:** 1000–2000mg timed releases 3x / day[99]

  Vitamin C helps protect your cells against the effects of free radicals. Free radicals are molecules that form when your body breaks down food. Free radicals form with tobacco smoke and radiation from the sun, X-rays or other sources. Free radicals might play a role in heart disease, cancer and other diseases.

- **B-complex vitamin**[100]

  B vitamins are important for ensuring the healthy functioning of body's cells. B Vitamins help the body convert food into energy. B Vitamins create new blood cells. B Vitamins maintain healthy skin cells, brain cells, and other body tissues.

- **Omega 3**: 2 grams twice daily[101]

Omega-3 fatty acids lowers inflammation.

- **Black Elderberry Extract** activates SIRT6. 1 teaspoon[102]

Elderberry has lots of antioxidants and vitamins that may boost your immune system. They could help tame inflammation, lessen stress, and help protect your heart, too.

- **Ubiquinone:** 100mg

Ubiquinone—also known as COQ10–supports mitochondria; improves NAD+/NADH ratio.

- **PQQ:** 20mg

PQQ Helps lower inflammation and improves mitochondrial health.

- **Urolithin A**: 500 mg

Urolithin A works with taurine and glutathione to renew the mitochondria.

- **Black Cumin**

Black Cumin has antiviral, antioxidant and anti-inflammatory properties. When you're congested black cumin helps open up your lungs. Its an antihistamine. Black Cumin can help get rid of a cough. All these are helpful properties in the fight against long COVID. Take 1 gram morning and evening.

- Melatonin

Melatonin is well known as a sleep aide. But did you know— that melatonin reduces inflammation in the body. Melatonin has antioxidant properties. That means melatonin can help protect cells from damage caused by free radicals. Free radicals are unstable molecules that can damage cells and cause inflammation. Damaged and inflamed cells contribute to chronic conditions. Chronic conditions give long COVID a home.

- **Sulforaphane:** take the mixed blend of myrosinase and glucoraphanin in 475–500 mcg doses[103]

Sulforaphane neutralizes toxins. Sulforaphane may reduce inflammation and improve heart health. Inflammation can help cause different kinds of cancer. Sulforaphane may reduce the risk of diseases of the nervous system. The most prominent of these is Alzheimer's disease. Sulforaphane reduces the area over which long COVID can gain linger.

You cannot take sulforaphane alone. It is not bioavailable. The stomach will break it down. You can take its precursors: myrosinase and glucoraphanin.[104] These two precursors working together[105]—will convert to sulforaphane.[106]

- **Taurine:** start with 3 grams @ day. After a month scale back to 1 gram @ day

Taurine improves brain and heart function. Taurine supports nerve growth. It lowers blood pressure and calms the nervous system. It supports energy metabolism. Taurine supports healthy gene expression. Taurine protects your cells against different types of stress.

- **Creatine Monohydrate:** take 3–5 grams daily

Creatine Monohydrate has been used for decades by the body building community to strengthen the muscles. In recent years creatine has been adopted by the longevity community because it firms up old muscles. It has anti aging effects. How does this happen? Creatine Monhydrate increases ATP production. That means that you'll have more energy. Creatine eases brain fog and fatigue issues.

Remove sugar from your life

There are different types of diets, including keto, carnivore, vegan, or pescatarian. They all have one thing in common. These diets help to cut sugar and refined carbs consumption.

Scientific literature is clear: sugar is what cancer feeds on.[107] Sugar causes type II diabetes and Alzheimer's disease. Sugar damages the cardiovascular system causing all manner of heart disease.[108]

Sugar depletes your body of Vitamin B, C, D, Magnesium, Calcium, Chromium, Copper, and Zinc.[109] Sugar degrades the innate immune system. Sugar makes the body vulnerable to Long COVID.

Follow these simple steps to reduce sugar in your diet:
- Clean your cupboards—remove candy, cookies, and other sugary snacks.
- Limit your fruit intake to berries.
- Learn to read labels—look at the sugar contents in the foods you eat. Aim for zero sugar.

- Check the sugar levels in your drinks from Starbucks. Smoothies and milkshakes can have hidden sugar levels. Again, aim for zero sugar.

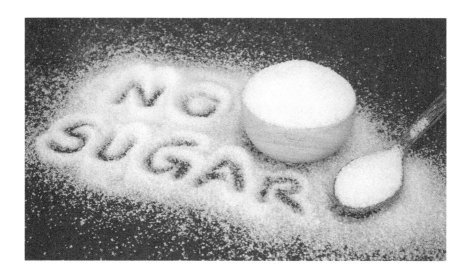

Avoid seed oils[110]

The Standard American Diet (SAD) contains many seed and vegetable oils. Industrial seed and vegetable oils undergo many stages of processing. These processes make them toxic to the body over time.

Seed and vegetable oils have too many Omega-6 fatty acids.[111] Our bodies were designed for a 1–1 ratio of Omega-6 fatty acids to Omega-3 fatty acids.[112] Americans eat too much seed and vegetable oil. Modern American diets boast an average omega-6 to omega-3 ratio around 10 to 1. These numbers can rise as high as 30 to 1. The standard recommendation for health is 4 to 1.[113] But centenarians will have an omega-6 to omega-3 ratio of close to 1 to 1.[114] Now that's something to consider.

Stop using vegetable and seed oils. Try to avoid them altogether. Over-heated and oxidized seed oils produce trans-fats and lipid peroxides as byproducts.

Higher-than-normal levels of polyunsaturated fats can reduce energy. These bad fats contribute to deadly inflammation in the body. Bad fats contribute to obesity, diabetes, and heart disease.

Consider eliminating these from your food:
- Canola oil
- Corn oil
- Cottonseed oil
- Grapeseed oil
- Rice bran oil
- Safflower oil
- Soy oil
- Sunflower oil

The oils below will help you:
- Extra virgin olive oil
- Extra virgin avocado oil
- Extra Virgin coconut oil

Improve Your Gut health

Your lower stomach is radically different from your upper gut. Your upper gut consists of the stomach and small intestine. Acids and enzymes digest food in the stomach and small intestine. These acids and enzymes come from pancreas and gall bladder. Your lower gut consists of the large intestine and the bowels. Bacteria digest food in your lower gut. No digestive juices are involved. 25–54 percent of the organic matter in healthy stools consist of living and dead bacteria. These bacteria provide many beneficial chemicals that your body needs to protect itself from disease. These chemicals are part of the innate immune system.

Prebiotics

The best way get a healthy gut is to feed the bacteria in your gut with resistant starches. Resistant starches are also known as prebiotics. These are starches that the digestive juices in your upper gut cannot break down.

Healthy stools look like Lincoln logs or torpedoes. If you don't have that look—there are some simple solutions.

Air pop popcorn. Popcorn is a low histamine food. Put some coconut oil on the popcorn. Coconut oil is a low histamine food. If you are not on a low histamine diet—you can also add olive oil. Then sprinkle in some nutritional yeast. Nutritional yeast has no histamine but it can trigger histamine in some products. (Every person has unique dietary triggers. Experiment.) Add salt, pepper, garlic and turmeric. They are all low histamine.

You can also make Keto Bread. Keto bread is full of resistant starches. Again, resistant starches do not break in down the upper stomach. Rather they become food for bacteria in your lower gut.

There are many recipes for Keto bread online. Just google "keto recipe". Take your pick.

Probiotics

You also want to bring new bacteria to your lower gut. Its healthier to have a large diversity of healthy bacterian in your lower gut.

Here's the rub. The best source of probiotics is fermented foods. Alas, fermented foods are high in histamines.

If you have histamine intolerance then you can't eat fermented foods. Don't eat fermented dairy products. Don't eat cheese (especially aged), yogurt, sour cream, buttermilk, and kefir. Don't eat fermented vegetables, such as sauerkraut, natto and kimchi.

Rather, take a probiotic pill that has a wide diversity of probiotic bacteria.

You may not have histamine intolerance. In that case eat all the different varieties of fermented foods that you can.

Add sunlight

We are not designed to live indoors like bats. Modern populations have been moving indoors since the first industrial revolution in 1840. That process has accelerated in the last 30 years. Spending extended hours indoors is unhealthy. A lifestyle without constant exposure to sunlight can set you up for illness and death. For example, 90 percent of people who die of COVID-19 have low Vitamin D levels.[115] Low Vitamin D is a direct result of lack of exposure to sunlight.

Our bodies need sunlight for optimal health.[116] It is important to get a at least one-hour of exposure to sunlight daily.

Why?

Your skin converts high frequency ultra violet sunlight into vitamin D.[117]

There's more.

The body makes melatonin in the pineal gland. The body also makes melatonin in the mitochondria of your cells. This happens when low frequency infrared light and near infrared light from the sun strike your body.[118] Near-infrared light penetrates deeper under the skin than infrared light. Near-infrared penetrates to the mitochondria of cells beneath the skin. The mitochondria are the powerhouses of the cell and the body. The low-frequency sunlight interacts with the mitochondria to create melatonin.[119]

This melatonin protects you from disease.[120]

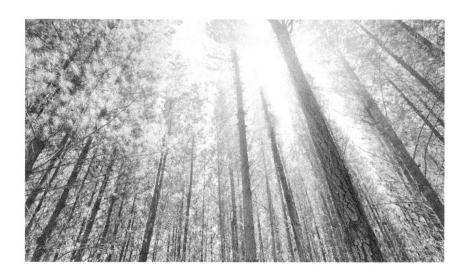

Melatonin, protects you from disease because in the mitochondria—melatonin creates glutathione.[121]

Glutathione is arguably the body's most important antioxidant in the body's innate immune system. Melatonin, through Glutathione, provides a primary defense weapon for the immune system.

There's more.

Sunlight makes the body make nitric oxide.[122] Nitric oxide is an important molecule in the body's innate immune system. The infrared and near-infrared spectrums of sunlight penetrate below the skin. There, they interact with the inner lining of the capillaries to produce nitric oxide. Nitric oxide is necessary for both men and women. Nitric oxide sustains your cardiovascular health.[123]

Capillaries are the smallest blood vessels in the body. Nitric oxide enables the blood vessels to expand and contract.[124]

This includes the big blood vessels and the little capillaries. This includes blood vessels coming from the heart, and blood returning to the heart. Big and small, coming and going, all blood vessels expand and contract with each pump of the heart. They do this with the help of nitric oxide created by capillaries in the presence of sunlight.

The body needs nitric oxide. Without nitric oxide, blood pressure increases. The blood vessels stiffen and crack. Bad things follow. The crack allows plaque to invade the arterial walls. This is the start of cardio vascular disease.

Getting out into the sunshine is more important than ever.

Studies have shown that exposure to more sunshine can help mitigate COVID-19 deaths.[125] For example, in England, Italy, and the USA, COVID-19 deaths were lower in summer than in winter. Similar studies show the same result in Europe and North America.[126]

COVID-19 is like seasonal flu in this respect because there is more sunlight in the summer than in winter. Seasonal flu like COVID stikes in the winter when people are not outside and the sun is low. As a result, during the winter, the body is not making enough vitamin D, melatonin, and nitric oxide.[127]

This reality is different for the people living near the equator. They tend to have much darker skin because there is so much sunlight. When they live near the equator their darker skin screens out the sunlight.[128] Their skin color is a natural sun tan lotion that absorbs less sunlight. So, their dark skin provides protection from the intense sunlight.

Things change when dark-skinned people move to the northern or southern latitudes. Their dark skin is no longer an advantage. Their dark skin prevents them from absorbing well the weak sunlight. To get their daily dose of Vitamin D, melatonin, and nitric oxide—they need more sunlight.[129]

People from northern Europe have lighter skin. This is because lighter skin absorbs the weaker sunlight in the northern hemisphere. So, light-skinned people need less of the northern sunlight. A little sunlight will give them their daily dose of Vitamin D, melatonin, and nitric oxide.[130]

Red light therapy[131]

There are alternatives to sunlight. You can get the low frequency infrared and near infrared light from red light therapy.

Sunlight consists of many different light spectrums. Red light therapy is a treatment that uses two of the sunlight spectrums. These light spectrums are low frequency infrared and near infrared. These frequencies improve skin appearance. They help your body create melatonin and nitric oxide.

You can also increase your nitric oxide levels with l citrulline.[132] Take 1 gram daily. You can also increase your melatonin levels by taking a supplement. Take 10 mg of melatonin before bed.

Heat and Cold

Your body does not need emotional stress. Your body does need physical stress. This is true on many levels. For now, we'll just talk about immune support.[133] Both heat and cold improve the body's immune system.

A simple way to do this is by contrast showers in the morning. Start your day with a hot shower. Then turn off the heat and turn on the cold. Go back and forth three times. You'll feel very frisky afterwards. Also, your immune system strengthens.

As mentioned before, don't do this until you have lowered your stress levels.

Another strategy is to go to your local gym. After a work out, spend 15 minutes in the sauna. If there is a swimming pool—take a dip in the pool. Go to the sauna either before or after you go swimming.

Again, don't do this until you have lowered your stress levels. You want your body to handle the physical stress. But without having the stress set off long COVID symptoms. We will point you to a tool later on that will enable you to track your stress levels.

Improve oxygen use

Deep breathing is a free option for improving the oxygen in the blood.[134] Deep breathing is an easy way to relax and let go of your worries.[135] You can do deep breathing anywhere; it only takes a few minutes. This process helps to ease stress and lower your blood pressure. Deep breathing increases oxygen levels and relaxes tense muscles. Other terms for this process are belly breathing, diaphragmatic breathing, and abdominal breathing.

Learning healthy ways to relax can help you avoid unhealthy choices. Stress makes it hard to make healthy choices. You can be more mindful when you're relaxed. More oxygen will clear the cobwebs from your mind and lighten your step.

Use this step-by-step guide to learn deep breathing exercises:[136]

1. Sit up straight in a comfortable position. You can be in a chair with your feet on the ground or sit cross-legged on the floor.

2. Put one hand on your stomach below your ribs and the other on your chest.

3. Breathe in through your nose, letting your stomach expand. The hand on your stomach should rise, while the hand on your chest should move very little.

4. Exhale through your mouth. Push the air out of your lungs and contract your stomach muscles. The hand on your stomach should move in as you exhale.

5. Repeat this pattern of breathing for 10 deep breaths.

You will feel more relaxed after a few deep breaths. If you're still feeling stressed, do 20 deep breaths. Remember, you can do this anywhere. You can do this anytime you need to relax.

Take a few minutes to focus on your breath. Breathe deep. Your mind becomes clearer, and your body feels lighter. You feel like you've finished a workout. Your blood now has more oxygen.

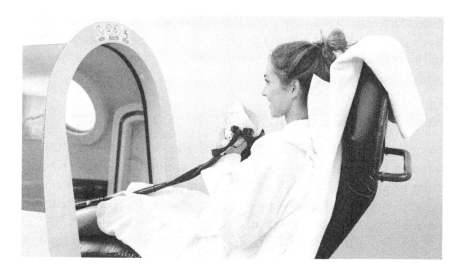

Hyperbaric oxygen therapy[137]

COVID-19 can cause low oxygen levels in the blood. Some people do not display shortness of breath but still, have low oxygen levels. Hyperbaric oxygen therapy is the solution for shortness of breath and breathing difficulty.[138]

Hyperbaric oxygen therapy is pricy. A home hyperbaric oxygen therapy machine costs $5,000 or more. At a clinic—a one-hour visit can cost $100–$400.

Long COVID sufferers may be able to go to their primary care doctor for a cheaper option. Ask your doctor for a referral to get hyperbaric oxygen therapy. This strategy may help you find hyperbaric oxygen therapy covered by insurance.[139]

After good exercise, your body will feel light and your mind will feel clear. In part, that's because your body enjoys high oxygen levels. The same thing happens after you have experienced hyperbaric oxygen therapy. Your body feels light. Your mind feels clear. Your body enjoys high oxygen levels. You experience the runners high without running.

Continuous Positive Airway Pressure (CPAP)[140]

Using a CPAP is another way of getting more oxygen into your body. This delivers air under pressure to your lungs while you sleep. These machines can cost $500, but you can get them free with insurance.[141] Go to your primary care doctor for a referral to a sleep clinic. This is especially important if you snore. But again, long COVID sufferers can have low blood oxygen levels. CPAP's will enable you to get proper rest because you're getting enough oxygen. You won't be exhausted in the morning.

Restore Your Taste and Smell

Some people experience a change to their taste and smell following COVID-19 infection. This abnormal sense of smell or taste goes by the name of parosmia. There are other variations. Hyposmia is the decreased sense of taste and smell. Anosmia is the loss of sense of smell. These changes in the ability to taste and smell are usually temporary. But in some cases, they can be permanent.

Olfactory retraining is the process of training your nose to smell. It involves smelling strong scents every day. These include citrus, cloves, eucalyptus, rose and lemon. You don't need to choose these scents. You can choose other scents. Choose the scents for which you have a strong memory. A convenient way to get these smells is by means of essential oils.

This is the strategy. Smell the essential oil scents while you remember what that scent smelled and tasted like. This helps to reconnect your nose and tastebuds with your brain. So in the future you will smell and taste lemons when you put your nose to lemon. Same goes for the other scents. Research has shown it can improve parosmia in long COVID patients.

Smell these substances for 15 seconds, twice a day for several weeks or several months. Olfactory retraining has been associated with significant improvements in the ability to taste and smell,

It often takes about 6 to 12 weeks to notice an impact and up to 24 weeks for maximal impact.

Intermittent Fasting

Fasting causes stress. You'll need to know how much stress you can handle before you attempt a fast. The next chapter will include instructions for obtaining a device. This device will help you track your stress levels.

That said, intermittent fasting reduces inflammation. Inflammation weakens the body. Inflammation enables COVID to get a foothold in the body. So fasting is another tool in your toolkit.

There are many different forms of fasting, each with its own potential benefits and risks. Some of the most common forms of fasting include:

- **Time Restricted Feeding.** This involves restricting food intake for certain periods of time. For example, only eating during an 8-hour window each day.
- **Alternate-day fasting.** This involves eating one day and fasting the next. On fast days you only eat about 500 calories or less. We don't recommend this as it can lead binge eating on non-fast days.
- **Water fasting.** This involves consuming only water and a multivitamin. Do this for a period of time, usually 1–3 days.
- **Long-term fasting.** This involves restricting food intake for several days or weeks. Consult with your doctor before you do this.

It is important to consult with your doctor before starting a fast. Fasting can have potential health risks. This is true for people with certain medical conditions. This is also true for people who are taking certain medications.

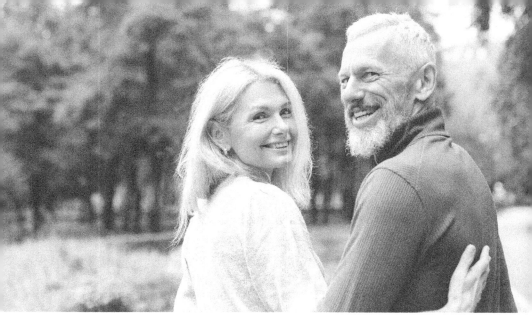

Chapter 3:
How to Manage Stress

This section will cover several options about mindset and alternative ways to heal. We will start with Dynamic Neural Retraining System.[142] This system uses a wearable monitoring device.

Dynamic Neural Retraining System™ (DNRS) is a new, drug-free, self-directed program that uses the principles of neuroplasticity.

Neuroplasticity is the idea that your brain can "rewire" itself.[143] Your brain can change its structure and function throughout your life. This change comes as a result of your experiences. This means you can retrain or rewire your brain if you like. This retraining or rewiring can help overcome many health issues. including trauma, chronic illness, and Long COVID symptoms.[144]

Neuroscientists once believed that the brain could not adapt after a certain age. They believed that the brain cannot change once a person reaches adulthood. New research has proved otherwise.

The DNRS program helps you change your brain's structure and function. DNRS retrains the brain.[145] "DNRS enables your body to move from a state of survival. Survival is characterized by fight or flight and freeze.[146]

Everyone understands fight or flight. That's what jacks up your adrenaline and cortisol. That's the source of stress. Sometimes the stress can be so high that a long COVID sufferer will freeze. They can't do anything.

You want to move to a new state. That state is the state of growth and repair. Growth and repair is where true healing can take place. The good news is that anyone can reverse the brain's over-sensitized "fight, flight, or freeze" mode.

DNRS helps to repair the neural pathways ravaged by stress. It does this by using brain-retraining techniques. The retraining solves a problem created by COVID. The brain can become so sensitized to COVID that it is reacting to COVID even when there is no cause. Why is this happening? The brain has been rewired by COVID to give you long COVID symptoms. DNRS rewires the brain back to its normal state. These techniques can rewire neural pathways and get you on the path to healing and growth.

Life will improve when you calm the nervous system. This will also regulate immune function and reverse chronic, post-viral illness.[147]

When you retrain your brain and nervous system, you reclaim your life. DNRS offers a safe, reliable way to shift your body from "fight, flight, or freeze" mode. The goal is to return to the mental state that enables healing, growth, and repair.

You can begin the DNRS online brain-retraining program through this link. You can become part of the community of recovered long-haulers.

Long COVID Monitoring Device

The most important thing you can do to avoid COVID symptoms caused by stress—is to pace yourself. You have to learn exactly how much you can do without setting off your symptoms.

Scripps Research is a nonprofit American medical research facility. Scripps created a health solution based on the principles of neuroplasticity.[148] They develop a wearable device that monitors a person's stress. This helps people to live within their stress limits. Stress triggers Long COVID symptoms. Using this device can help prevent overstressing yourself.[149]

This device has a feature called "body battery." The "body battery" transforms your health by using verifiable data. It logs your sleep, your stress levels, and your activity. The device uses these data to measure your "heart rate variability".[150]

The wearable device gathers information throughout the day and night. The device generates a percentage score from your activities.

A Long COVID sufferer can keep track of their score throughout the day and night. The score measures your stress levels and establishes an upper limit for stress. This upper limit is the most stress you can tolerate without setting off long COVID symptoms. The generated data helps you to know when to stop and rest. You can rest before your activity triggers Long COVID symptoms.

This is especially helpful when you want to get into an exercise program or begin to do hot and cold therapy. You can check your stress levels and stay within your limits.[151]

The downside

This device may cause issues for people sensitive to EMFs (Electromagnetic fields). If you are using Fitbit and other similar devices, you won't have a problem using this device.

Go to https://www.facebook.com/groups/longcovidproblemsandsolutions/ to participate.

Mindset and Long COVID

Realizing that you have Long COVID can be disheartening. Especially when you know Long COVID issues can be lifelong. This reality can trigger negative feelings and make you depressed. When you have bad feelings, let them flow. Fighting negative feelings can make things worse. Allowing the feelings to flow helps you to overcome them.

This is a medical issue and not a psychological one. To overcome this feeling, open your laptop. Type what you feel. Put your negative emotions into words. Write your stressors, including anger and bitterness. Write other related feelings connected to Long COVID. Write everything that comes to you.

If that does not help, you can cry when your emotion pushes you to tears. Crying is a great way to release negative emotions. Cry for as long as it takes to get those feelings out.

Mindset is very important. The thoughts you choose can either fill you with hope or make you miserable.

Mindset problem is a new disease affecting many people. If you try everything in this book, you can improve your chances of getting relief. Its especially helpful to stack one treatment on another.

Remember that feelings like anger, sadness, and hopelessness are normal. These feelings only last 40–60 minutes at a strong, intense level.

- If you feel hopeless and sad, it will pass. It's cathartic.
- Do not feel scared. Let the feelings pass.

Allowing your negative feelings to flow improves your mental health.

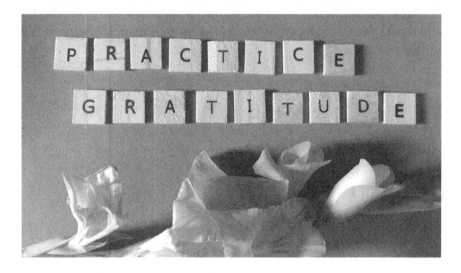

Practice the Attitude of Gratitude

Science shows that gratitude actually change changes your mind. Gratitude improves your attitude. Practicing gratitude gives you the fastest relief from negative self-talk. The two forms of thought cannot cohabit in your mind at the same time. Push yourself to continuous thoughts of gratitude. The negative self-talk will go away.

How do you do this?

Notice what you can be grateful for. It could be the little things. The air you breathe. The food you eat. It could be the sound of music or the silence. It could be your home or a distant star. Cultivate a an attitude of gratitude about your situation. This, in turn, changes how you think. Gratitude changes how you behave in the moment. It helps to develop a supportive and life-affirming habit for the future. Gratitude is a proactive means of engaging in the here and now. Gratitude makes for a positive attitude. You need a positive attitude to heal.

Self Help Options

Self-help books and videos are important for your life. You can start now if you haven't read any self-help books or listened to any self-help videos on YouTube. They can help you to manage your life better. A better-managed life is one with lower stress. You can create the life that you want regardless of your condition.

Stop Bad Habits, Create Good Ones

It would be great if you could break bad habits and develop good ones. In "Atomic Habits", James Clear[152] explains how to do this. He explains how it's not your fault for not being able to develop good habits. He said you lack the proper systems to support breaking bad habits—or developing good habits.

Do you want to break bad habits and create good habits? James Clear's book "Atomic Habits" will help you.

These are excerpts from "Atomic Habit" on how you can build good habits and break bad habits:

- A simple way to build a good habit is to make it easy and visible.
- A simple rule for breaking a bad habit is to make it hard and invisible.

For example, if you love chocolate and want to break the bad habit of eating too much chocolate, keep it out of sight. Make it difficult to get the chocolate. If you want to eat more apples, put them on the kitchen counter where they are easy to grab.

It is more important to build habits and stick to the habit. For example, if you want to build a good habit like walking every day—it doesn't matter how far you walk at first. What matters most is that you walk. Walk any distance. Walk to the end of your driveway. Walk the length of your block. Walk to the front door of your building.

Some people tend to push themselves too hard. This will create a problem. We set high standards for the first attempt. Then we become disappointed when we fail. Instead, create mini-habits. Habits that are very easy to complete.

Consistency builds confidence and inspires you to do more. When your walk is consistent, you will have a growing desire to do more. When you are in the mood, take advantage of the good mood to do more. Some days, you won't be able to walk to the driveway. That's great too. The important thing is to keep up the good habit.

The College of London did a study on how long it takes to create a good habit. They found that it takes an average human 66 days to create a good habit.

Most of us may think that it takes only 21 or 30 days. The study showed that it takes much longer. Also, there is variability. It only took 10 days for some people to develop good habits. And for others, it took over 250 days!

Developing good habits takes time. Some people develop good habits faster than others. So, don't give up if it takes you longer than others.[153]

Buy the book "Atomic Habits" by James Clear to help you navigate your self-improvement. Read it and read it again. Keep rereading the book in the morning. Just a page or two will do. You'll find that just reading the book will make you feel optimistic. Why? Because the book makes you aware of your daily habits. The book shows you how you can change your habits on a day to day basis.

Good habits lower stress.

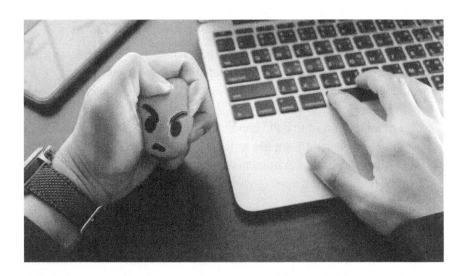

How to Get Things Done (Without Stress)

There are many things that you can do to manage stress. Making your bed is a great way to start a good day. People consider it insignificant, but it can put your day in the right direction. At night, always set up for your morning routine.

If you have a more complex life, learn to manage yourself better.

Consider.

Our minds are like Random Access Memory (RAM). RAM is a temporary memory bank where your computer stores data it's currently working on. RAM keeps data accessible so that it can retrieve it when needed.[154]

You can open a limited number of browsers on a computer. Your computer slows down when there are too many open tabs and applications. Go beyond that, and your computer freezes. People have similar characteristics. We become slow when we have many things going on. Our ability to perform slows down.

Like a computer's RAM, our memory cannot handle too many open "applications" and "tabs".[155] We are not designed to keep track of too many things at once. This can increase the stress level. It's worse for Long COVID sufferers.

How do you solve the problem of memory overload?

Consider.

When you go on vacation — what happens? The months and weeks before your vacation, you make lists of what to do. Then, you knock off everything on the lists. You do this so that while you're on your vacation, you don't have to think about anything but enjoying yourself. You do all you can to reduce stress while on vacation.

Imagine having this kind of relaxing activity all the time.

David Allen wrote the book "Getting Things Done: The Art of Stress-Free Productivity".[156] In this book, David Allen provides priceless lessons. It has become one of the most influential business books of all time. The acronym GTD (Get Things Done) is now even shorthand. It is a new way to approach personal and professional tasks. There are lots of websites and organizational tools developed around it.

This book shows you how to create an outer mind for yourself. One that you can rely on at all times. The outer mind is so reliable that you can always count on it. The outer mind enables you to trust what you're doing. You trust too in what you're not doing. Because you have all the elements of your to-do list written down. You have things set up so that you always know what to do and when to do it. You always have your priorities in line. The book shows you how to do this both for your personal life and your business life.

You don't do more than one thing at a time. You don't multitask. Rather, you do one thing after another. David Allen says that people who adapt to his practices enter a state called The Zone." The zone is a state of absolute focus where athletes are at their peak performance. David Allen calls this state: "Mind like water."

This practice is more complex than list making. Getting Things Done (GTD) is a system for managing stress-free productivity. It helps you create a catalog of reminders and weekly reviews.

You are free from having to remember tasks and to-dos. This can help you to focus on the task at hand—without stressing over what you're not doing. You're not overwhelmed by other things you need to remember.

Processing too much information produces stress. Try to process too much information and you become immobile. Information bounces around in your head. But you don't move.

Too Much Information (TMI) makes it harder to decide what to do. GTD eliminates stress by showing you what to do at the right time in the right place with the energy you have.

Master Getting Things Done (GTD) and your stress level at work and home will fall.

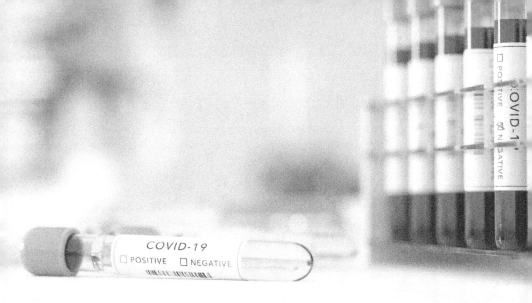

Finale

This book includes many current understanding and practical treatments. These treatments can decrease Long COVID symptoms. Work through each section of the book and give yourself time to heal. Understand your symptoms. Knowing what you are dealing with will help you to focus on how to proceed.

When COVID-19 started, no one knew there would be a long-term impact. People undergo months of monitoring. It took thousands of brave people to disclose their health issues and concerns. Many of them received poor treatment. Doctors told them it was "in their head". They instructed them to find a therapist.

Long COVID is not in your head. It is real. You are feeling a real illness taking over your body.

This book seeks to help you to take control of your health.

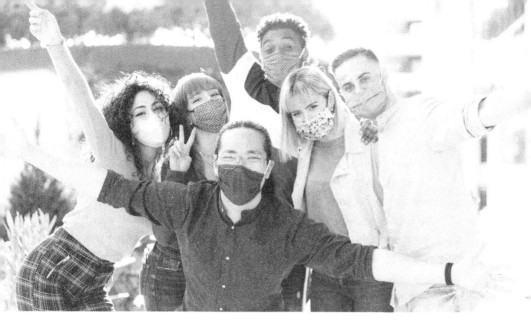

Conclusion

We have given you many actionable solutions. Take the steps forward. Each step leads to another step which leads to better health.

At the beginning of this book, we talked about what to do first. Test and treat for histamine intolerance. Then we talked about the body and its' innate immune system. Many of us have frail immunity. COVID-19 preyed on those frailties and settled in to take over. The goal is to try different treatments to restore the strength of your innate immune system. Our innate immune system becomes stronger when given the proper treatments.

For most of the book we talked about lowering stress. Stress is what most often sets off the worst symptoms of long COVID.

Long COVID Healing Checklist

We have provided a checklist for you. This will help you to navigate each section. Focus on your health, keep track of what you have completed, and concentrate on your success.

Use this checklist to check your progress every month. It can help you track your progress and identify your failures. Tracking your progress can help you to prevent further failure. You can adopt lifestyle changes and work to feel better.

Track what you do, how you feel and changes in your symptoms. You can mark improvements and changes as you follow the road to better health from Long COVID!

Date: _____

Months you contract COVID: _____

COVID Symptoms:

Make a list of the symptoms you have now. Refer to Index The Symptoms of Long COVID

_____ _____ _____

_____ _____ _____

_____ _____ _____

_____ _____ _____

Antihistamine: Date started _____ Date ended: _____

Did you feel better? _____

What changes did you notice? _____

Low Histamine Diet

Food removal start date: _____

What changes did you notice? _____

Food addition

Food added: _____ Start Date: _____ Symptoms: _____

Food added: _____ Start Date: _____ Symptoms: _____

Food added: _____ Start Date: _____ Symptoms: _____

Supplements (Chapter 2)

Name: _____ Date started: _____
How do you feel? _____

_____

Name: _____ Date started: _____
How do you feel? _____

_____

Name: _____ Date started: _____
How do you feel? _____

_____

Stress Reduction

In what ways did you reduce stress this month (check all that apply)
_____ Meditation
_____ Self-hypnosis
_____ Prayer
_____ Friends
_____ Walk outside
_____ Pet
_____ Reduce news input

Health Support options (check those that apply)

_____ Removed/reduced sugar
_____ Increased time in the sun
_____ Hot/Cold Therapy
_____ Hyperbaric 02 Therapy
_____ Deep Breathing

What positive changes have you noticed this month?

_____
_____
_____
_____

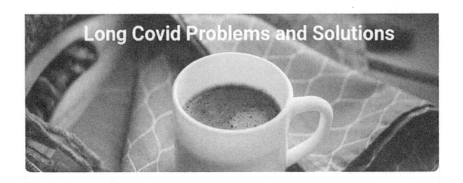

Long Covid Problems and Solutions

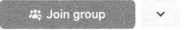

Join the evolving conversation about your symptoms at **Long COVID Problems and Solutions** (https://www.facebook.com/groups/longcovidproblemsandsolutions/).

Endnotes

1   How Many People Have Long COVID? The Statistics Are 'Pretty Scary'

2   Is long COVID a new autoimmune disease?

3   Post-COVID Conditions (e.g. Long COVID)

4   Long COVID or Post-COVID Conditions

5   Guidance on "Long COVID" as a Disability Under the ADA, Section 504, and Section 1557

6   Long COVID: Over 200 symptoms, and a search for guidance

7   50 percent of people who survive COVID-19 face lingering symptoms, study finds

8   Estimates of long COVID are startlingly high. Here's how to understand them

9   What We Know About Long COVID So Far

10   Histamine intolerance and long COVID

11   Long COVID or Post-acute Sequelae of COVID-19 (PASC): An Overview of Biological Factors That May Contribute to Persistent Symptoms

12   Psychological distress before COVID-19 infection may increase risk of long COVID

13   Do antihistamines help with Long COVID symptoms?

14   Do you need a low histamine diet?

15   NAD+ in COVID-19 and viral infections

16   Endogenous Deficiency of Glutathione as the Most Likely Cause of Serious Manifestations and Death in COVID-19 Patients

17   Mast cell activation symptoms are prevalent in Long-COVID

18   Mast cell activation syndrome and the link with long COVID

19   Mast cell activation syndrome

20   Mast Cell: A Multi-Functional Master Cell

21   What is the difference between IgE allergies and mast cell triggers? Can you have IgE allergies and mastocytosis? Are there tests to identify these triggers?

22   The Role of Mast Cells in the Defence against Pathogens

23   What is a DAO Deficiency? How to Increase DAO Enzymes Naturally

24   What Are Histamines?

25   Histamine Intolerance—Signs, Symptoms & Treatment Options

26   Pathophysiology of Post-COVID syndromes: a new perspective

27   Autoimmune response found in many with COVID-19

28   Histamine Intolerance: The Current State of the Art

29   Low-Histamine Diet

30   Elimination Diet

31   Histamine Intolerance

32   Why choose low-histamine foods?

33   Caution advised with low histamine diets for Long COVID

34   What Is Histamine Intolerance?

35   6 Natural Antihistamines to Help With Allergies

36   What is DAO? Diamine Oxidase Supplements Explained

NOTES

NOTES

NOTES

NOTES

NOTES

Made in the USA
Las Vegas, NV
02 May 2024

89406451R00046